RELAXTOCLARITY.COM

# Chiropractic Care for Clearer Vision
## Backed by Actual Case Studies

Dr. John DeWitt
9/28/2015

This book contains over 15 research studies describing how chiropractic care has helped restore clearer vision in patients suffering from a variety of maladies.

## Table of Contents

Chiropractic Care for Clearer Vision .................. 9
    Vitalism ................................................................. 10
    Naturalism ... ......................................................... 11
    Spiritualism ... ....................................................... 12
    Subluxation .......................................................... 14
About Me .................................................................. 17
RESEARCH SOURCES OUTLINE ............................. 21
    Visual Recovery Following Chiropractic Care ................................................................................ 22
    Symptomatic Arnold-Chiari Malformation and Cranial Nerve Dysfunction: A case study of applied kinesiology cranial evaluation and treatment .............................................................. 24
    Irlen Syndrome, Headaches, Dyslexia and Other Visual Disturbances ..................................... 30
    Visual Recovery Following Chiropractic Intervention .......................................................... 32
    Changes in Visual Acuity in Patients Receiving Upper Cervical Specific Chiropractic Care ...... 36
    Strange Bedfellows – Chiropractic and Vigabatrin ............................................................. 41
    Obstacles to research in complementary and alternative medicine .............................................. 44
    Case Study: Improvement in Meniere's Disease, Balance, Coordination & Quality of Life Following Network Spinal Analysis Care 47

Vision, the Cervical Spine and Chiropractic ...50

Recommended Clinical Protocols and Guidelines for the Practice of Chiropractic ....52

Improvement in Vision in a Patient with Diabetic Retinopathy Following Network Spinal Analysis Care .................................55

Gestational Diabetes Mellitus...........................59

Vision: Your Neurological Window...................60

Post-Concussion Patient Care: Relevance of the Chiropractic Adjustment ...............................62

Improved Immunity and Vision: Chiropractic Testimonials ................................................66

Quality of Life Improvements and Spontaneous Lifestyle Changes in a Patient Undergoing Subluxation-Centered Chiropractic Care: A Case Study ..............................................................68

Cerebral Dysfunction: a theory to explain some of the effects of chiropractic manipulation ....71

Visual Recovery from Diplopia in a 13-Year-Old Following Chiropractic Intervention...................75

Treatment of severe glaucomatous visual field deficit by chiropractic spinal manipulative therapy: A prospective case study and discussion......................................................81

ADDITIONAL STUDIES...............................91

The types and frequencies of nonmusculoskeletal symptoms reported after chiropractic spinal manipulative therapy........92

Changes in eyesight associated with upper cervical specific chiropractic .................................. 95

Changes in eyesight associated with upper cervical specific chiropractic .................................. 97

Subluxation location and correction ................. 99

The eye, the cervical spine, and spinal manipulative therapy: a review of the literature.................................................................. 100

The prospective treatment of visual perception deficit by chiropractic spinal manipulation: a report on two juvenile patients ....................................................................... 102

The step phenomenon in the glaucomatous recovery of vision with spinal manipulation: A report on two 13-year-olds treated together. .................................................................................. 103

Bilateral simultaneous optic nerve dysfunction after pariorbital trauma: Recovery of vision in association with chiropractic spinal manipulation therapy. ........................................... 104

Monocular scotoma and spinal manipulation: the step phenomenon. ......................................... 106

Effects of a chiropractic adjustment on changes in pupillary diameter: a model for evaluating somatovisceral response. .............. 108

Study on cervical visual disturbance and its manipulative treatment. ........................................ 110

Monocular visual loss after closed head trauma: immediate resolution associated with spinal manipulation ............................................... 111

Chiropractic adjustments and esophoria: a retrospective study and theoretical discussion. ................................................................................ 113

The side effects of the chiropractic adjustment ................................................................................ 114

The Treatment of Presumptive Optic-Nerve Ischemia by Spinal Manipulation ...................... 116

Monocular visual loss closed head trauma: immediate resolution associated with spinal manipulation. ............................................................ 117

An observer's view of the treatment of visual perception by spinal manipulation. A survey of 16 patients ................................................................ 119

Cortical blindness, cerebral palsy, epilepsy and recurring otitis media: A case study in chiropractic management. ................................... 120

Case report: spinal strain and visual perception deficit ..................................................... 124

# Chiropractic Care for Clearer Vision

**Introduction:** The history of chiropractic began in 1895 when **Daniel David Palmer** of Iowa performed the first chiropractic adjustment on a partially deaf janitor, **Harvey Lillard,** who then mentioned a few days later to Palmer that his hearing seemed better. This led to Palmer opening a school of chiropractic two years later. The word "chiropractic" was coined from Greek root words by Rev. Samel Weed. Chiropractic's early philosophy was rooted in…

## Vitalism…

*Vitalism is a scientific doctrine that "living organisms are fundamentally different from non-living entities because they contain some non-physical element or are governed by different principles than are inanimate things". Where vitalism explicitly invokes a vital principle, that element is often referred to as the "vital spark" or "energy", which some equate with the soul.*

## Naturalism...

*In philosophy, **naturalism** is the "idea or belief that only **natural** (as opposed to **supernatural** or **spiritual**) laws and forces operate in the world." Adherents of naturalism (i.e., naturalists) assert that natural laws are the rules that govern the structure and behavior of the natural universe, that the changing **universe** at every stage is a product of these laws*

## Spiritualism…

*Spiritualism (philosophy), the idea that there exists an immaterial reality that is beyond the reach of the senses*

…and other constructs that were not amenable to the scientific method. Chiropractic's founder, D.D. Palmer, attempted to merge science and metaphysics. In 1896, D.D. Palmer's first descriptions and underlying philosophy of chiropractic was strikingly similar to Andrew Still's principles of osteopathy established a decade earlier. Both described the body as a "machine" whose parts could be manipulated to produce a drugless cure. Both professed the use of spinal manipulation on joint dysfunction/subluxation to improve health.

## Subluxation

*A spinal subluxation is when the vertebrae are misaligned with the other neighboring vertebrae thus creating pressure on the spinal nerves. Initially, these misalignments are just that…spinal misalignments, but when the pressure on the spinal nerves is enough to effect the organ systems, muscles and other joints…THAT is when it becomes a subluxation.*

Palmer drew further distinctions by noting that he was the first to use short-lever High Velocity Low Amplitude (HVLA) manipulative techniques using the spinous process and transverse processes as mechanical levers.

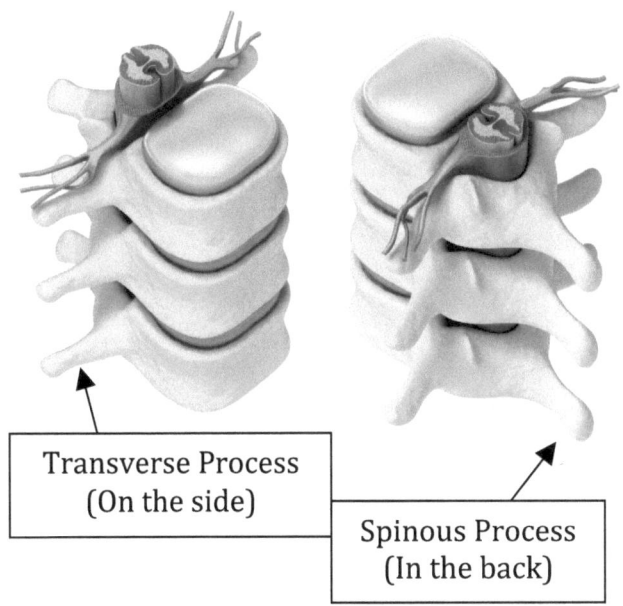

Transverse Process (On the side)

Spinous Process (In the back)

He described the effects of chiropractic spinal manipulation as being mediated primarily by the nervous system. The nervous system is the master system. It controls every system, organ and cell in the body. It just makes sense that having a better connection to the nervous system is going to mean a healthier organism...AKA YOU!

# About Me

I am a Vanderbilt University graduate who earned a full athletic scholarship after my first semester. I went on to become the starting defensive end for the next four years and was awarded The Wade Looney Award for outstanding work ethic. I continued my football career with the NFL Houston Oilers, NFL Europe Champion Scottish Claymores, Montreal Alouettes of the CFL, San Francisco Demons of the XFL, and several teams in the AFL including three seasons with the LA Avengers.

After retiring from football, I earned my Doctor of Chiropractic degree from Los Angeles Chiropractic College. I practice in Orange County, at Bergman Family Chiropractic, specializing in sports nutrition golf injuries, natural vision correction and corrective chiropractic care.

I am an active volunteer for the Assistance League of Newport-Mesa, the Lili Claire Foundation and supporter of Boys Town of California. I can be seen on the Healthy OC segment of the Real OC on KOCE hosted by Heidi Cortese.

I have been happily married to Cathy DeWitt for over 17 years. We live in Irvine with our two adorable dogs, Murphy and Maggie.

I started wearing glasses in the $8^{th}$ grade and suffered with the hastle of them for decades. Contacts were no better but a necessary evil for me while I played football. I came across the Bates' Method after years of searching for a natural alternative. I went on to write *You Don't Need your Glasses or Contacts: natural Solutions for Clearer Vision without Drugs or Corrective Lenses,* and *20 Surprising Foods for Clearer Vision* prior to writing this book on the benefits of chiropractic adjustments in regards to vision.

I am not a certified Bates' Practitioner but rather a student of life that knows the body is built to be healthy. Given the proper hydration, nutrition, movement and inner peace, all of us should live to be 120 or more!

I wrote this book for the misinformed people out there that think chiropractic is an "alternative therapy" at best. My hope is that the research outlined in these pages will show that a corrective chiropractor is the first person to be considered when someone isn't feeling well and/or has the desire to live life at their best!

There is a considerable amount of chiropractic and medical terminology which I tried to minimize as much as possible.

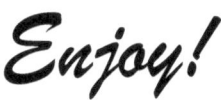

# RESEARCH SOURCES OUTLINE

This outline is organized in alphabetical order by the last name of the author. Page numbers in parenthesis follow notes when appropriate.

## Visual Recovery Following Chiropractic Care

A. *Visual Recovery Following Chiropractic Care*.

Curl, D. Dynamic Chiropractic, Vol. 10, Issue 4 (1992).

- Provides a brief review of chiropractic literature focused on **spinal manipulation and visual improvements**. Research by author was conducted through *Chirolars*, the only full operational chiropractic computerized database.

- Cites Bryant et al., as support for the use of cervical manipulation for the treatment of oculomotor palsy.[1]

---

[1] See Gilman G, Bergstrand J. Visual recovery following chiropractic intervention. California Chiropractic Association Journal, pp. 22, 26, 28 (1990).

- Cervical manipulation has facilitated visual improvement because often visual disorders have often been reported in conjunction with degenerative changes to the cervical spine.

## Symptomatic Arnold-Chiari Malformation and Cranial Nerve Dysfunction: A case study of applied kinesiology cranial evaluation and treatment

B. *Symptomatic Arnold-Chiari Malformation and Cranial Nerve Dysfunction: A case study of applied kinesiology cranial evaluation and treatment.* Cuthbert, S., Blum, C. Journal of Manipulative and Physiological Therapeutics, Vol. 28, No. 4, pp. 289.e1-6 (2005).

- Case report of a young woman with complex optic nerve neuritis that was exacerbated by an Arnold-Chiari malformation (ACM) type I of the brain (289e.1). ACM "is a projection of the medulla and cerebellum that extends through the foramen magnum and into the cervical spinal canal (289e.1).

- Patient was a 20-year-old female with "retrobulbar neuritis (optic nerve neuritis) of the right eye, as diagnosed by her general practitioner, ophthalmologist, and a neuroradiologist, reported that she had gone blind in her right eye 11 days earlier and was markedly frightened. She stated that everyone's face had suddenly gone blank to her upon awakening one morning" (289.e3). Three months preceding vision loss the patient was in an automobile accident.

- During patient's initial examination "she could only detect outlines of large objects and specific colors with her right eye. With her left eye covered, she could not detect the presence of the Snellen eye chart on the wall. She revealed an example of the ocular lock phenomenon, with saccadic motion in both eyes. Almost every angle of her gaze exhibited disorganization in the movement of the 2 eyes, or see-saw nystagmus, a common finding in ACM cases" (289.e3).

- Patients diagnosed with ACM deal with corticospinal and sensory deficits, along with cerebellar signs and lower cranial nerve palsies (289e.1).

- ACM has been known to cause developmental defects of the skull bones, spinal column, meninges and spinal cord.

- Evidence exists supporting the use of chiropractic care as a form of treatment for ACM.[2]

- The differentia diagnosis of the patient's visual problems was conducted through the use of applied

---

[2] See Murphy DR, Goldstein D, Katz M. Chiropractic adjustment to the cervical spine and the Arnold-Chiari malformation. J Manipulative Physiol Ther 1993;16:550 – 5 and Smith JL. Effects of upper cervical subluxation concomitant with a mild Arnold-Chiari malformation: a case study. Chiropr Res J 1997;4:77 - 81.

kinesiology (AK) cranial and cranial never testing procedures (289.e2). Via AK testing procedures patient was diagnosed with cranial faults, which eventually resolved following chiropractic treatment (289.e5).

- Patient received oculobasic correction in order to improve the dural tension upon the coccyx, which was accompanied by the integration of the visual reflexes with the pelvic-righting reflexes (289.e3). For the term oculobasic, "Oculo" relates to the visual0rughting reflexes, while "basic" refers to the Logan Basic technique for sacral and spinal treatment/manipulation (289.e3).[3]

---

[3] See Goodheart GJ. Applied kinesiology 1979 workshop procedure manual. Detroit (Mich)7 the author; 1979. p. 24 – 6, and Coggins WN. Basic technique: a system of body mechanics. Creve Coeur (Mo)7 ELCO Publishing Company; 1983. p. 77 - 85.

- Patient underwent AK and sacro-occiptal chiropractic techniques, which utilize cranial bone dysfunction and manipulative strategies (289.e4) and reported the following improvements/outcomes: "After each cranial correction, eye movements were retested, and less saccadic motion and ocular confusion were noted. The cranial corrections were continued at the initial office visit until her eyes were moving through the cardinal fields of gaze smoothly and equally. At the end of the first treatment, the patient noted that she could see the author's (S.C.) face through her right eye as well as her mother's face who was sitting approximately 10 ft across the room. She was then taken to a Snellen eye chart and was able to read 20/30 vision with her right eye. On her second visit 2 days later, she had 20/20 visual acuity. There was still some reported blurriness with reading fine print, but she reported that every day since her first correction, she was seeing with greater clarity" (289.e3).

- By patient's third visit her visual acuity had reached 20/13, and she no longer reported blurriness with reading, and vision continued to improve on each follow-up visit (289e.4)

- The patient's cranial faults diagnosed through AK testing procedures appeared to resolve after treatment.

## Irlen Syndrome, Headaches, Dyslexia and Other Visual Disturbances

C. *Irlen Syndrome, Headaches, Dyslexia and Other Visual Disturbances*. Floto, J. Dynamic Chiropractic, Vol. 27, Issue 03 (2009).

- The headaches that chiropractors treat are often caused by scotopic sensitivity syndrome, also known as Irlen syndrome, which is a hereditary and permanent condition characterized by visual disturbances that cause difficulties in functioning and reading.

- Often young people who suffer from Irlen Syndrome are wrongly placed in special education programs and exhibit behavioral issues because of their disability.

- Article argues that chiropractors should be aware of Irlen Syndrome in order to deliver patient's with the relevant chiropractic adjustment and other treatments in order to improve vision and other Irlen Syndrome symptoms.

## Visual Recovery Following Chiropractic Intervention

D. *Visual Recovery Following Chiropractic Intervention.* Gilman, G., Bergstrand, J. Journal of Behavioral Optometry, Volume 1, Number 3, pp. 73-74 (1990).

- Case study of elderly man who reported complete loss of vision following a head trauma. Patient underwent postsurgical correct vision acuity along with cataract removal and intraocular lens implantation (73).

- Patients head trauma caused after falling "between two logs and hit both sides of his head. He immediately experienced head pain and dizziness. The following day he awoke he had lost all vision"(73).

- Optometrist diagnosis indicated mild macular degeneration and bilateral slight optic atrophy, and client was unable to respond to traditional vision tests (73).
- At the time of patient's original optometric examination, it was determined that optometric treatment would not benefit patient, who was subsequently referred to a chiropractor because both authors of the case study had already seen patients who had experienced improved vision changes after receiving chiropractic adjustments (73).
- Following chiropractic treatment patient had a vision examination and reported that vision improvement began following his third chiropractic adjustment (74). Patient reported being able to read better, at first stating that vision improved so that he first began to see shades of grey, instead of just

black, and then following several additional adjustments, there was an addition of blue swirling circles and yellow areas in the field of gray. Following these improvements patient began to distinctly see actual light coming through a window (74).

- Two theories for patient's visual improvement as a result of chiropractic adjustment:

a) Chiropractor Mabel Palmer's theory that "an anatomical communication between the spinal nerves of the upper cervical region and the various visual fibers." (74). Chiropractic manipulation may have eliminated the physical interference with the nerves causing diminution of visual functions, resulting in the return of patient's visual function (74).

b) By eliminating the innervational intervention caused by the cervical soft tissue trauma to the head, the optic nerve blood supply could have returned to normal after its previous constriction caused by the head trauma.

## Changes in Visual Acuity in Patients Receiving Upper Cervical Specific Chiropractic Care

E. *Changes in Visual Acuity in Patients Receiving Upper Cervical Specific Chiropractic Care*. Kessinger, R., Boneva, D. Journal of Vertebral Subluxation Research, Volume 2, No. 1 (1998).

- Case study investigating the relationship between Upper Cervical Specific chiropractic care and changes in visual acuity (1). This longitudinal study is concerned with upper cervical specific care in order to investigate "the relationship between frequency of adjustments (hence presence of vertebral subluxation) and changes in visual acuity among a population of subjects previously naïve to any form of chiropractic (3).

- The study's duration of investigation "was designed to assess the concept of restoration of function as opposed to changes due to a short term stimulus-response evoked by a given force application to the spine" (3).

- Study Criteria: "required that participants (1) had no prior Upper Cervical Specific Care, (2) maintain their current lifestyle, (3) commit to following the chiropractic plan of care designed for the study. Consecutively, from the first 100 new patients entering care during the period of August through October, 1996, sixty seven met the requirements" (3)

- Characteristics of Case Population: "The population under study represented sixty seven subjects who had not previously experienced chiropractic care. They ranged in age from 9 to 79 years, averaging 46.4 ± 17.0. The subject group consisted of 37 females (48.7 ± 18.9 years) and 30 males (43.5 ±15.7 years). They were evaluated for each eye, before and six weeks after receiving chiropractic care, relative to their ability to accurately identify letters in a standard Snellen Chart." (1).

- Significant literature supports the association between head/cervical neck trauma and visual disorders in both the absence and presence of degenerative joint changes (1).

- Professionals have noted the intimate relationship between the autonomic nervous system and the eye, and evidence indicates that there is a link between somatovisceral eye responses and vertebral subluxation (2).

- Vision returned in a different study of a patient whose optometric and ophthalmological examinations revealed only a visual response to be bilateral light perception, after eleven C1 adjustments over a three month period, at a follow up examination the patient reported being able to ready normally, and all subsequent ophthalmic findings supported a return to vision (2).

- In this study, vision acuity was measured as a function of the correct identification of letters in each distance category (3), and both eyes were compared before chiropractor treatment, and then again 6 weeks following care (4).

- The studies suggests that Upper Cervical Specific (C-1, C-2) chiropractic care caused a differential improvement in the visual acuity of both eyes, as measured as the percentage change in vision acuity before and 6 weeks after chiropractor care (5)

- Through upper cervical chiropractic adjustment procedures employed within the current study, vision acuity improvements appear to be linked to the correction of vertebral subluxation and chiropractic methods of upper cervical specific care.

## Strange Bedfellows – Chiropractic and Vigabatrin

F. *Strange Bedfellows – Chiropractic and Vigabatrin*. Gorman, RF. Dynamic Chiropractic, Vol. 19, Issue 19 (2001).

- This article focuses on the interaction between medicinal drugs, chiropractic and vision improvement, while also presenting the theory of tunnel vision information (TVI). TVI is the theory that vision improves when the spine is manipulated.
- Author also posits "spinal manipulation changes neurological function, and by so doing, allows the body to use innate resources to heal general bodily ills".
- The author along with other practitioners have discovered that a specific type of visual field loss known as concentric constriction of the visual fields

was associated with spinal derangement, and that the visual abnormality can be immediately recovered if the spine is manipulated in a nonspecific way.

- In a different study the researchers directly addressed the use of chiropractic treatment finding that the recovery of vision could occur via outpatient chiropractic adjustments, though such recovery was quicker when anesthesia was used.[4]

- Also focuses on the use of Vigabatrin and other drugs for the treatment of epilepsy that often (30% of the time) cause complications that result in irreversible contraction of the visual fields (4).[5]

---

[4] See Stephens D, Mealing D, Pollard H, Thompson P, Bilton D, Gorman RF. Treatment of visual field loss by spinal manipulation: A report on 17 patients. *JNMS* 1998:6(2) pp 53-66.

[5] See Eke T, Talbot JF, Lawden MC. Severe persistent visual field constriction associated with Vigabatrin. *BMJ* 1997:314, pp. 180-1.Schmitz B, Jokiel B, Schmidt TK, et al. Visual field defects under treatment with Vigabatrin, carbamazepine and

Cites studies that illustrate how the specific feature of a neurological illness such as epilepsy (ie. constricted visual fields), can be immediately resolved by chiropractic spinal manipulation.

---

valproate; a prospective study. *Epilepsia* 1999:40 (Suppl. 2.) p. 257. Kalvianinen R, Nousianen I, Mantjyarvi M, Riekkinen Sr. P. Absence of concentric visual field defects in patients with initial tiagabine monotherapy. *Epilepsia* 1999:40 (Suppl.2.) p. 259. Lawden MC, Eke T, Degg C, et al. Visual field constriction associated with Vigabatrin treatment. *Epilepsia* 1999:40 (Suppl.2.) p 257.Update on visual field constriction with Vigabatrin. *Aust Adv Drug Reactions Bull*1999:18(3).

## Obstacles to research in complementary and alternative medicine

G. *Obstacles to research in complementary and alternative medicine*. Gorman, RF. Medical Journal of Australia, Vol. 180 (2004).

- The author RF Gorman provides a defense for his argument that chiropractic treatment can lead to visual improvements in appropriate patients. This thesis/argument has not been completed accepted, especially by the Australian medical community, of which Mr. Gorman is a member as an ophthalmologist (95). Medical Journals such as this one have not accepted Gorman's arguments " because randomised controlled trials have not been performed."(95).

- Gorman's description of his much-cited 1992 study is contained below:

" In 1992, I [RF Gorman] sent 12 consecutive patients demonstrating constricted visual fields to four senior fellows of the then Royal Australian College of Ophthalmologists. The patients were examined by those consultant scrutineers, who agreed that the visual fields were constricted in all occasions. The patients were seen at independent locations, and I was present only on one occasion. The patients were then treated by spinal manipulation under anaesthesia, with immediate recovery of the visual fields being noted on wakening from anaesthesia. This recovery of vision merely reiterated many earlier anecdotal demonstrations. In every case, the scrutineers agreed that the vision had recovered when, at an independent location subsequent to the treatment, they saw the patients"(95).[6]

- In another study Gorman, along with other authors provided outpatient chiropractic spinal adjustments for 17 patients. The entire population reported immediate improvements to their visual fields; computerised static perimetry was used to measure these improvements (95).[7]

---

[6] See Gorman RF. The treatment of visual perception defect by spinal manipulation: a prospective peer-reviewed study of twelve consecutive patients. 24th Annual Scientific Congress of the Royal Australian College of Ophthalmologists. 1992 Nov 1-6; Sydney. 3. Langford-Wilson A. New view of tunnel vision. The STAR (Mt Isa) 1982; 14 Sep. 4. Howarth J. Claims of answer to vision scourge. The NT News (Darwin) 1982; 13 Nov: 17. 5. Morrison J. A dangerous twist. 60 Minutes. TCN Channel 9, NSW, 22 Jun 1986.

[7] See Stephens D, Mealing D, Pollard H, et al. Treatment of visual field loss by spinal manipulation: a report on 17 patients. J Neuromusculoskeletal Sys 1998; 6: 53-66.

## Case Study: Improvement in Meniere's Disease, Balance, Coordination & Quality of Life Following Network Spinal Analysis Care

H. *Case Study: Improvement in Meniere's Disease, Balance, Coordination & Quality of Life Following Network Spinal Analysis Care*. Kemp, A. Feeley, K. Annals of Vertebral Subluxation Research, pp. 107-119 (Nov. 2013).

- Though this case study does not specifically address visual improvements as a result of chiropractic, it does provide an explanation of the practice of Network Spinal Analysis (NSA) and how it has positive effects for multiple non-musculoskeletal issues including vision improvement (109), stating that:

"Although NSA does not claim to be a cure for medical conditions, it is estimated that more than 12,000 patients currently receive NSA care and there are many reports of improvements in symptoms of medical conditions.18, 21, 22 To our knowledge there have been no reports of NSA care and Meniere's disease; however, there have been reports of NSA care and positive effects with multiple non-musculoskeletal issues"

- This case study follows the treatment of a 56 year old male being treated a chiropractic clinic, who complained of:

" bilateral carpal tunnel symptoms, numbness in both feet after sitting, and pain and fullness in the left ear .... accompanied by dizziness and progressive hearing loss experienced over the past twenty years. Physical examination revealed significant structural and neurological imbalances. Spinal subluxations were identified at multiple levels of the spine" (107).

- On patient's 89th adjustive visit, which occurred one year and 9 months into regular chiropractic treatment, patient completed a re-evaluation questionnaire, within which patient noted improvements in vision, mood, sleep and overall comfort (109).

- One of the case study doctor's concluded that the chiropractic treatment that patient underwent was subsequently followed by afferent somatic information that created changes in the vestibule-cochlear system which produced patient's positive changes in hearing. The cortical integration of visual, somatic and vestibular information influenced this afferent somatic information (111).

## Vision, the Cervical Spine and Chiropractic

I. *Vision, the Cervical Spine, and Chiropractic.* Kent, C. The Chiropractic Journal (1996).

- Article provides an outline/review of the primary literature on chiropractic treatment for visual improvement. Outlines the comprehensive review conducted by Gorman and Terrett in 1995, within which spinal manipulation and adjustment was conducted and followed by changes in patients intraocular pressure, oculomotor function, pupillary size and visual acuity.[8] These studies involved a broad age population and chartered visual improvements, returns to normalcy and higher qualities of life for an assortment of patient's after little as one spine treatment from a chiropractor.

---

[8] See Terrett AGJ, Gorman, RF. The eye, the cervical spine, and spinal manipulative therapy: a review of the literature. Chiropractic Technique, vol. 7, no. 2, p. 43 (1995).

- Patient's in the Gorman studies suffered from a variety of visual impairments including monocular vision loss, monocular vision defects, accompanied with headaches and other physical complaints.

- Article makes the important note that though chiropractic is not a treatment for esophoria, blindness, or scotoma, the correction of vertebral subluxations provides patients with benefits such as visual improvements that are not are not directly with their musculoskeletal complaints. Ultimately even non-specific chiropractic interventions have the potential to bring about favorable results with regards to visual issues.

## Recommended Clinical Protocols and Guidelines for the Practice of Chiropractic

J. *Recommended Clinical Protocols and Guidelines for the Practice of Chiropractic*. The International Chiropractors Association (2000).

- The guidelines contain an examination of peer-reviewed literature that relate to the use of chiropractic treatment for non-musculoskeletal disorders (251).

- Outlines Gillman and Bergstrand's study of an elderly male with traumatic vision loss, where in optometric and ophthalmologic examinations revealed that there was no appropriate conventional treatment (252). Within this article the authors noted that "behavioral optometrists have often been interested in the work of chiropractors and the resulting vision changes."[9]

- Literature from Schutte, Tesse and Jamison, is briefly discussed. This retrospective review involved 12 children suffering from exophoria, a form of heterophoria in which the eyes have a tendency to deviate outward, concluding that these patients could respond to cervical spinal adjustments (252).[10]

- The connection between positive effects from chiropractic cervical manipulation was indicated by the report from Changjiang et al regarding 114 cases of patients who presented both cervical

---

[9] See Gilman G, Bergstrand J. Visual recovery following chiropractic intervention. Journal Behavioral Optometry, vol. 1, no.1, pp.73-74 (1990).

[10] See Schutte B, Teese H, Jamison J: Chiropractic adjustments and esophoria: a retrospective study and theoretical discussion. Journal of Australian Chiropractic Association, Vol. 19, No. 4, pp.126 (1989).

spondylosis and visual disorders (252).[11] In 83% of the cases visual improvement was noted in 83% of the cases, and out of 54 of the cases that the researches followed up on for a minimum of six months, 95% of the population illustrated a stable therapeutic effect. Also contained within this report were cases of vision being returned to blind eyes (252).

---

[11] See Changjiang I, Yici W, Wenquin L, et al. Study on cervical visual disturbance and its manipulative treatment. Journal of Traditional Chinese Medicine (1984).

## Improvement in Vision in a Patient with Diabetic Retinopathy Following Network Spinal Analysis Care

K. *Improvement in Vision in a Patient with Diabetic Retinopathy Following Network Spinal Analysis Care.* Irastorza, M., Knowles, D., Knowles, R. Diabetic Retinopathy. Annals Vertebral Subluxation Research (2012).

- Case study tracking the "reorganization and reduction of intraocular pressure (IOP) in a chiropractic patient with diabetic retinopathy and concurrent loss of vision undergoing Network Spinal Analysis (NSA) care (25).

- The goal of this case study was to address "the normalization of intraocular pressure (IOP) in a diabetic patient with diabetic retinopathy and concurrent loss of vision using NSA care. During a three year period of NSA care, the IOP pressure decreased and normalized."(26).

- The patient was a 46-year-old male with Type 1 insulin dependent diabetes (25).

- Patient suffered from diabetic retinopathy (DR), which is the worldwide number one cause of preventable blindness in adults (25).[12] Patient reported that his progressive vision loss in both eyes was the result of diabetic retinopathy (26). Vision loss had commenced 2 years before NSA treatment, and he suffered from a right eye optic nerve that had poor circulation (26).

-Advanced DR causes blindness and vision loss, more specific consequences include "vitreous hemorrhages, neovascular glaucoma (NVG),

---

[12] See Resnikoff N, Pascolini D, Etya'ale D, et al. Global data on visual impairment in the year 2002. Bull World Health Organ 2004; 82: 844-51.

tractional retinal detachment, and/or vision loss"(25).[13]

- Patient received NSA care 221 times during a 3-year period and "Network protocol was administered sequentially through three levels of care"(27). Each visit's NSA treatment involved "a low force contact on specific spinal gateway region, relative to the level of care and phase of AMCT [Adverse Mechanical Cord Tension] presenting in the patient."(27).

- After three months of treatment that patient's retina specialist stated "the retina was re-attaching to the eye contributing to his vision coming back" (27).

---

[13] See Simo R, Carrasco E, Garcia-Ramirez M, Hernandez C. Angiogenic and antiangiogenic factors in proliferative diabetic retinopathy. Curr Diabetes Rev 2006; 2: 71-98.

- Following 8 months of chiropractic treatment, patient began reporting seeing colors and shapes in his left eye for the first time in 5 years (25). Patient also reported a drop in his intraocular pressure (25).
- Case study asserts that there could be a potential link between NSA chiropractic care and the subsequent normalization and decrease of intraocular pressure of the retina (28).
- The clinical goal of NSA is to address sympathetic tone by reducing and self-regulating the vertebral subluxation, and reorganization of neural and spinal integrity (28). Case study infers a connection between NSA resulting in increased neural and spinal integrity, along with the decrease of spinal subluxation patterns, providing a positive effect on the sympathetic nervous system (28).

## Gestational Diabetes Mellitus

L. *Gestational Diabetes Mellitus.* Marriott, CL. Journal of Clinical Chiropractic Pediatrics, Vol. 11, No. 22 (2010).

- Article provides more background about diabetes and its symptoms as they relate to vision complications (789).
- Diabetes is characterized by a chronic dysfunction of the metabolism that is characterized by hyperglycemia.
- Long-term hyperglycemia is characterized by damage, eventual failure and long term dysfunction of an assortment of organs including the eyes
- Blurred vision is a characteristics of marked hyperglycemia.

## Vision: Your Neurological Window

M. *Vision: Your Neurological Window*. Masarsky, C. Dynamic Chiropractic, Vol. 23, Issue 25, 2005.

- Article briefly discusses that the spinal nerves play a very important role in vision, because the "Nerves from the cervical spine (neck) and upper thoracic spine (the upper back) help to dilate (widen) the pupil - the opening that allows light into the eye."
- These spinal nerves also make distance vision possible by helping change the shape of the lens, while also controlling the blood vessel wall muscles that supply the brain and the eyes.
- Chiropractic treatment often focuses on correcting misalignments/fixations (subluxations) in the upper thoracic spine and cervical spine which can disturb the same spine nerves that affect vision.

- Argues that chiropractic adjustments to correct subluxations can help alleviate the related visual disturbances. In support of this argument, the author cites a study conducted by a Missouri chiropractic research team who "reported that even some people with 20/20 vision at their first visit have better than 20/20 vision after two weeks of chiropractic care."[14]

---

[14] See Kessinger R, Boneva D. Changes of visual acuity in patients receiving upper cervical chiropractic care. *Journal of Vertebral Subluxation Research* 1998;2(1):43.

## Post-Concussion Patient Care: Relevance of the Chiropractic Adjustment

N. *Post-Concussion Patient Care: Relevance of the Chiropractic Adjustment.* Masarsky, C. Dynamic Chiropractic, Vol. 32, Issue 15 (2014).

- Discusses the use of chiropractic adjustment in the treatment of concussion manifestations including vision, vestibular function and vision deficits.

- Vision dysfunction is a common symptom of concussions and other head trauma.

- Article cites the Gilman and Bergstrand case study of an elderly man who suffered from a head injury and became completely blind the day after the head trauma. Examination by an ophthalmologist and optometrist supported patient's claim of blindness because both examinations revealed and absence of a pupillary response.

- After being followed for three months without a return of vision or recovery of the pupillary response, a chiropractic examination was subsequently conducted. Chiropractic conducted the following treatment:

"The chiropractor found a C1-C2 fixation on motion palpation. He adjusted the patient's upper cervical spine 11 times over a period of three months. After the third adjustment, the patient was able to perceive light. After the 11th adjustment, the patient could see rays of light coming through a window, could distinguish different colors, and demonstrated a normal pupillary response. After another two months of chiropractic care, the patient was able to read."[15]

---

[15] See Gilman G, Bergstrand J. Visual recovery following chiropractic intervention. *Chiropr: J Res Chiropr Clin Invest*, 1990;6:61-63.

- Article also references a 2012 Sweat and Pottenger study regarding a 75-year-old woman who suffered from a concussion following a slip-and-fall injury that had occurred 10 years earlier. At the time of initial chiropractic treatment, patient complained of a lazy left eye that interfered with reading. Upon examination:

"Chiropractic physical and X-ray examination findings were consistent with upper cervical subluxation. Extraocular muscle examination revealed a strabismus, characterized by the left eye lagging behind when the patient was asked to look to her right. She was unable to walk heel-to-toe, instead using a wide stance to ambulate."

- Patient received chiropractic treatment 22 times over a period of less than year. By the end of this treatment, patient reported that though left eye control was not perfect, patient's left eye control had improved and she no longer had problems with reading for as long as she wanted. Patient reported:

"improvement in extraocular muscle function, she also noted improvements in the brightness, clarity and color perception of her vision. These improvements began shortly after the first adjustment and progressed during this period of follow-up.[16]

---

[16] Sweat R, Pottenger T. Seizure, ataxia, fatigue, strabismus and migraine resolved by precise realignment of the first cervical vertebra: a case report. *J Upper Cervical Chiropr Res*, 2012 Mar 12:20-26.

## Improved Immunity and Vision: Chiropractic Testimonials

O. *Improved Immunity and Vision: Chiropractic Testimonials*. Pathway Magazines, (2010).

- Testimonial of parent whose son reported vision problems and trouble reading. Optometrist believed this issues caused by a "tracking issue that made it difficult for him to focus on anything, especially close up".
- Parent began taking son for chiropractic treatment, seeing the chiropractor three times per for week for adjustments. These visits gradually decreased over time due to Eric's improvement
- Child began demonstrating noticeable changes in sports ability, school and reading.
- The original optometrist that the child had been seeing for 2 ½ years conducted another examination

after chiropractic treatment began. This optometrist reported positive changes to the child's eyes and stated that "If Eric were seeing me for the first time today, I would not prescribe glasses for him."

## Quality of Life Improvements and Spontaneous Lifestyle Changes in a Patient Undergoing Subluxation-Centered Chiropractic Care: A Case Study

P. *Quality of Life Improvements and Spontaneous Lifestyle Changes in a Patient Undergoing Subluxation-Centered Chiropractic Care: A Case Study*. Pauli, Y. Journal of Vertebral Subluxation Research, pp. 1-9 (2006).

- This case study involved a 36-year-old male who presented health problems including "stress, headaches, eye pain and 14 years left leg pain radiating to the foot with subjective loss of strength and sensation (2).

- Upon patient's first chiropractic examination he was diagnosed vertebral subluxation and adverse mechanical cord tension. The initial care plan included an adjustment schedule of three appointments a week for two months, and then for the next two months adjustment visits twice a week. Following the first five months of treatment, patient's adjustment schedule was reduced to once a week for a remaining two months (3).

- In relevant parts, patient's chiropractic treatment included:

"Adjustive care consisted, in various sequence and timing, of Network Spinal Analysis low force touch contacts, Torque Release Technique Integrator instrument, pelvic drop piece adjusting and Diversified structural high velocity, low amplitude adjustments to the aforementioned vertebral subluxations. Thermal and sEMG scan re-evaluations were performed at 4 weeks (12 visits), 8 weeks (24 visits), 14 weeks (36 visits), 26 weeks (52 visits) and 42 weeks (56 visits). After week 26, the schedule was spaced by constantly adding one additional week to reach monthly visits. Scans are to be taken every three months to monitor the patient's neural integrity." (3)

- Following the initial six-month period of chiropractic treatment, patient reported a self-rated 95% improvement in his left leg pain, eye pain and headaches (4). This improvement occurred gradually, he reported a 30% improvement following 12 visits, a 50% improvement following 24 visits, and a 60% improvement following 36 visits (4).

- In addition to reporting less physical pain, patient also reported that his overall quality of life had increased and reported less family-related and work-related stress as a result of his decreased pain and increased feelings of well being (4).

## Cerebral Dysfunction: a theory to explain some of the effects of chiropractic manipulation

Q. *Cerebral Dysfunction: a theory to explain some of the effects of chiropractic manipulation.* Terrett, A.G.J. Chiropractic Technique, vol. 5, no. 4 pp. 168-173 (1993).

- Presents the theory of brain hibernation as a possible explanation for how spinal manipulation as a mode of action to treat extremely difficult to quantify complaints such as visual disorders (168). This theory of brain hibernation as a potential explanation for many of the desirable effects of spinal manipulation was first presented by the medical practitioners Eric Milne and Frank Gorman (168).

- Gorman's book "Chiropractic medicine for rejuvenation of the mind" charted Milne's original use of spinal manipulation for the treatment of headaches. However, Milne eventually discovered patient's commenting that other health complaints such as tiredness, dizziness and glare distress had all been relieved following spinal manipulation (168).[17]

- Author posits that "a decrease in cerebral blood flow (CBF) could possible cause parts of the brain to "hibernate" (168). Both Milne and Gorman proposed that many people suffered from decreased brain functioning as a result of decreased CBF (169). The blood flow restriction to the brain is a result of the vertebrae being misaligned or malfunctioning, resulting in stress on the vertebral arteries that causes a constriction of the lumen (169). When the CBF is below a critical level, the

---

[17] See Chiropractic medicine for rejuvenation of the mind. Gorman, RF. Academy of Chiropractic Medicine (1983).

cells do not function, though they are still present (169).

- Changes in visual acuity, visual disorders and headaches are some of the signs and symptoms that have been theorized to cause decreased CBF, which is the result of decreased cerebral functioning (169).

- Provides an analysis of a private study conducted by Gorman of 12 patients who underwent spinal manipulation for visual disorders (170).[18] Gorman used four ophthalmologist who were all asked to examine patients both before and after treatments through the use of standard opthalmoscopic assessment methods. The vision improved, either in visual acuity or the visual field for all patients

---

[18] See An observer's view of the treatment of visual perception deficit by spinal manipulation: A survey of 16 patients. Gorman, RF. Published Privately (1991).

(170). Extracts from six of these reports can be located here on p. 170.

## Visual Recovery from Diplopia in a 13-Year-Old Following Chiropractic Intervention

R. *Visual Recovery from Diplopia in a 13-Year-Old Following Chiropractic Intervention*. Tymms, G. Journal of Clinical Chiropractic Pediatrics, Vol. 12, No.1, pp. 876-878 (2011).

- This case study focuses on the correction of over convergence and the resolution of apparent double vision following chiropractic manipulation (876).

- Patient was a 13-year old boy who suffered from intermittent diplopia (double vision) who was referred to chiropractic care by his optometrist. As a result of chiropractic intervention patient reported full resolution of symptoms are only one chiropractic treatment session along (876). Patient's double vision diplopia had already presented a year earlier and occurred on weekly basis (876).

- Diplopia is an eye condition where a single object appears as two objects, and the patient's case of binocular diplopia that was the result of accommodative insufficiency and convergence insufficiency. Accommodative insufficiency is the inability to focus/sustain focus at near distance, while convergence insufficiency is when the eyes have a tendency to drift outward wen focused on reading or other close work (876).

- Patients pre-chiropractic optometrist examination revealed:

"
- normal unaided visual acuity
- normal eye health, healthy optic nerves and fundi right & left
- normal pupil responses
- no significant refractive error
- normal near point of convergence (8cm)

- difficulty clearing a -2D focusing demand on normal print
- binocular eye co-ordination findings within normal range for age, with only mild over convergence at near distance when given a focusing demand of -2D" (877).

- Optometrist concluded that though there was a mild focusing issue, there was no ophthalmic cause for patient's double vision and a referral was made to a chiropractor.

- Patient's initial chiropractic examination revealed "normal cervical range of motion, unremarkable cranial nerve and upper limb neurological examination. Multiple areas of vertebral dysfunction were identified, specifically at C1, C2, C6, mid-thoracic, L4 and bilateral sacroiliac joints.

Muscle hypertonicity was noted in the rhomboid musculature bilaterally" (877).

- Patient's treatment involved "rotary and lateral thrusts to the cervical spine, followed by posteroanterior dorsal spine manipulation and manipulation of the lumbopelvic spine via an activator adjustment tool in the line of the correction. The patient reported full resolution of symptoms after 1 visit. He was seen on 2 more occasions over a 2 week period whereby by the 3rd visit it was ascertained that the vertebral dysfunction in the neck had corrected" (877).

- What makes this case study unique is the fact that the pre and post chiropractic treatment was performed in conjunction with an independent optometric evaluation (877). Patient's optometrist noted visual improvements following chiropractic treatment.

- Author's theories for why chiropractic treatment improved patient's diplopia (877):

    • Chiropractic adjustments remove neural impairments to the internal carotid artery and the abducens, trochlear, oculomotor and ophthalmic nerves.

    • Chiropractic care facilitates cervical subluxation affecting the sympathetic innervation to the blood vessels of the optic nerve.

    • Chiropractic care facilitates vertebral subluxation causes a reduction in vertebral artery flow resulting in neuronal ischemia to the occipital lobes.

- Provides an analysis of Gorman's "step phenomenon" which is the argument that recovery from a visual disturbance is a gradual process with different stages. This visual recovery is the result of a gradual increase of oxygen to inactive ischemic tissues (877). Support for this phenomenon is the case study of a 53-year old woman who suffered from loss of vision following a facial fracture resulting from a fall. Gorman and his co-authors were eventually able to "quantify multiple areas of cerebral ischemia from a single photon emission computerized tomography. However this was not re-performed post chiropractic treatment after the patient's vision had returned (877).[19]

---

[19] See Stephens D, Gorman RF, Bilton D. The step phenomenon in the recovery of vision with spinal manipulation: a report on two 13-yr-olds treated together. J Manipulative Physiol Ther 1997; 20(9):628-33.

# Treatment of severe glaucomatous visual field deficit by chiropractic spinal manipulative therapy: A prospective case study and discussion

S. *Treatment of severe glaucomatous visual field deficit by chiropractic spinal manipulative therapy: A prospective case study and discussion.* Wingfield, B. R. et al. Journal of Manipulative & Physiological Therapeutics, Vol. 23, Issue 6, pp. 428–434 (2000).

- Though scientific literature has long reported that visual disturbances are caused by musculosketal disorders of the cervical spine, what has not been reported until this case study is the tracking/use of spinal manipulative therapy (SMT) in a patient with clearly identifiable and specific ocular pathology ie. optic disk atrophy (428).

- Case report about a "25-year-old uniocular female patient with congenital glaucoma sought chiropractic treatment for spinal pain, headache, and classic migraine" (428). Loss of vision was nearly complete and accompanied by advanced optic disk cupping. This damage to the optic disk is caused by terminal glaucomatous damage (428).

- Patient's vision was severely impaired due to xanthogranuloma of the iris, which caused both a hemorrhage into the anterior chamber of the eye (congenital left hyphema) and an abnormal enlargement caused by raised intraocular pressure (IOP) (429). Xanthogranuloma is a benign and rare tumor that was located in the both eyes of the patient shortly after her birth (429). The xanthogranuloma tumor in the right was removed via radiotherapy, but the xanthogranuloma in the left iris persisted causing the eye to be removed when the patient was 3 years of age, and replaced with a prosthesis (429).

- Despite medical interventions and ongoing medication, the patient's glaucomatous process continued to rapidly progress, destroying patients peripheral vision, and by the age of 16, the patient was declared legally blind (429).

- Due to patient's extreme ocular pathology vision improvement as presumed to be extremely unlikely (429).

- Patient's chiropractic treatment began as a 2-week course of SMT chiropractic, with 4 treatments during the first week, and three treatments during the second week (430).

- Immediately following the first adjustment, patient reported significant visual improvement in her remaining eye and maximal vision improved was reported after 1 week and four chiropractic adjustments. These results were confirmed by an independent rexamaination reported by the patient's regular ophthalmic surgeon.

- Treatment involved "chiropractic SMT applied to the intervertebral segments listed as having chiropractic subluxation. Various specific spinal manipulative maneuvers were used according to the discretion of the treating chiropractor. All manipulations were manual, low-amplitude, high-velocity moves (diversified chiropractic technique). Most chiropractic SMT maneuvers resulted in a joint cavitation sound. The exact segments manipulated varied slightly from one treatment to the next, depending on palpatory findings on the day. Some muscle stretching and gentle trigger point–type soft-tissue manipulation were also applied to help facilitate manipulation. No anesthesia, sedation, or any other form of medication was involved in the intervention." (430)

- The positive outcome of this treatment was tracked via Goldmann perimetry and ophthalmic examinations of corrected visual acuity were performed immediately after and before each SMT chiropractor treatment. There was no more than 20 minutes between the commencement and completion of treatment and the subsequent eye exams (431).

- Following the first session of chiropractic surgery, patient reported vision improvement, including improved clarity in her inferior temporal field, and her total area of visual field (original 2%) had expanded to 11%, and eventually expanded to 20% by the end of her chiropractic treatment (431).

- The second session also produced visual field improvements, and visual fields continued to improve with treatments over the 4 sessions of the first week (431). In fact, examination via Goldmann perimetry illustrated that patient's total area of visual perception had increased from patient's baseline before treatment of 2% to approximately 20% of the normal field of vision. Patient's corrected visual acuity improved from 6/12 to 6/9 (431).

- Immediately after the "second session of chiropractic manipulation, the wedge of vision in the inferior temporal field had increased further to encompass most the quadrant.". Author posits that this illustrates the Stephens et al., step effect/phenomenon of the recovery of vision with spinal manipulation.[20]

- After the initial 2 weeks of treatment, the decision was made to continue chiropractic treatment as a supportive means to maintain visual and musculosketal improvements (431).

- Slight step effects continued to be recorded and the overall stabilization of the visual field was maintained, and monthly supportive SMT chiropractic treatment was effective in maintaining patient's visual field (431).

- As a result of the treatment, patient reported ability to more effectively enjoy and engage in

---

[20] See Stephens D, Gorman RF, Bilton D. The step phenomenon in the recovery of vision with spinal manipulation: a report on two 13-yr-olds treated together. J Manipulative Physiol Ther 1997; 20:628-33.

everyday activities with an independence not previously experienced.

- Ultimately, patient reported vision improvement within minutes of chiropractic therapeutic intervention following a period of over 10 years of visual deterioration that was subsequently followed by approximately 2 years of documented stable baseline vision (432).

- Chiropractic SMT removed sympathetic irritation, improving optical and retinal nerve head perfusion, and restoring electrical activity in previously hibernating neurons and/or axons (433). Author presents two explanations from these visual improvements resulting from the SMT chiropractic treatment (433). These two explanations arguably brought about visual improvement on their own, and/or in combination with one another. Author believes that the site of neurological functional improvement believed to cause the vision improvement was either an ocular phenomenon or a cerebral phenomenon (433).

- Improvement to patient's migraines accredited to the fact that those suffering from migraines often present an increased incidence of visual field loss, and migraines have also been linked to the same type of glaucomatous optic nerve damage experienced by patient (433).

- Ultimate case finding: "The improvement of this patient's vision after chiropractic SMT suggests a cause-effect relation. We have hypothesized that the presence of chiropractic subluxation in the cervical spine was responsible for irritating the cervical sympathetic nerves, thereby causing the cephalic episodic vascular irritability (ie. migraine) against a background of vascular spasticity (ie. interictal migraine)"(433).

# ADDITIONAL STUDIES

## The types and frequencies of nonmusculoskeletal symptoms reported after chiropractic spinal manipulative therapy

A. *The types and frequencies of nonmusculoskeletal symptoms reported after chiropractic spinal manipulative therapy.* Leboeuf-Yde C, Axen I, Ahlefeldt G, et al. J Manipulative Physiol Ther Nov/Dec 1999:22(9) 559-64.

-The goal of the study being reported by this source was to determine:

"How frequently [do] patients report nonmusculoskeletal symptomatic improvements and [what are] the types of such reactions that patients believe to be associated with chiropractic…"

- The test population consisted of: 20 consecutive patients from 87 Swedish chiropractors. The patients answered questionnaires at every return visit completing a total of 1,504 questionnaires. Out of these study, 23% of patients reported improvement in nonmusculoskeletal symptoms following their chiropractic treatment. These improvements included:

- "Easier to breathe (98 patients)
- Improved digestive function (92)
- Clearer/better/sharper vision (49)
- Improved circulation (34)
- Less ringing in the ears (10)
- Acne/eczema better (8)
- Dysmenorrhoea better (7)
- Asthma/allergies better (6)
- Sense of smell heightened (3)
- Reduced blood pressure (2)
- Numbness in tongue gone (1)
- Hiccups gone (1)

- Menses function returned (1)
- Cough disappeared (1)
- Double vision disappeared (1)
- Tunnel vision disappeared (1)
- Less nausea (1)"

## Changes in eyesight associated with upper cervical specific chiropractic

B. *Changes in eyesight associated with upper cervical specific chiropractic.* Kessinger, Robert. Pub. In Chiropractic Research Journal, Vol. 5, No.1, Spring 1998.

- A study was conducted on 65 patients in the private chiropractic office setting to assess the influence of upper cervical specific chiropractic care on eyesight.

- Subjects' eyesight was examined via Snellen Eye Chart with standard testing procedures.

- A before and after studies were performed as part of a six-week program of upper cervical specific chiropractic care. The study included patients who had no previous history of specific chiropractic care and were eight years old and older. Significant objective changes in eyesight were indicated by the study.

## Changes in eyesight associated with upper cervical specific chiropractic

C. Changes in eyesight associated with upper cervical specific chiropractic. Kessinger, Robert. Abstracts from the 14th annual upper cervical spine conference Nov 22-23, 1997 Life University, Marietta, Ga. Pub. In Chiropractic Research Journal, Vol. 5, No.1, spring 1998.

- Case study of a pediatric patient, a 17-year-old girl who suffered from glaucoma and chronic sins infections.

- Patient was born with her glaucoma and had undergone 13 separate eye surgeries before she was 15 months old.

- Girl began chiropractic adjustment treatment, one month before she was scheduled for adenoid surgery. Patient's chiropractic treatment including adjustment via the use of an hand held adjustment instrument, and craniosacral techniques were also performed. The results from this treatment are as follows:

"Two months prior to seeking chiropractic care she was placed under general anesthesia to get intraocular pressure readings of 21 in the right eye and 28 in the left eye. After one month of chiropractic care her intraocular pressure was measured as 17 R and 15 L. Patient's adenoid surgery was cancelled. After 4 months of care, the intraocular pressure was 14 R and 11 L. As of the writing of this paper the subject is 3 years old, is seen every two to four months and rarely has a cold or flu symptoms. Her intraocular pressure is normal and she is off all medications."

## Subluxation location and correction

D. *Subluxation location and correction*. Goldman, S. D.C. Today's Chiropractic July/August 1995 p.70-74.

- Case study no. 3 is about a 77-year old female patient who was diagnosed with ocular myothenia (blurred vision and double vision symptoms), by a neuro-ophthalmic specialist.

- The chiropractic treatment used focused on axis subluxation and by the 9th visit all symptoms of blurred and double vision had disappeared. The patient stayed under maintenance care and no recurring problems relating to these vision issues was reported.

**The eye, the cervical spine, and spinal manipulative therapy: a review of the literature.**

E. *The eye, the cervical spine, and spinal manipulative therapy: a review of the literature.* Terrett, A.G. and Gorman, R. Frank. Chiropractic Technique Vol. 7, No. 2, May 1995.

- Gorman, an ophthalmologist, and Terret, a chiropractor, decided to write an article together in order to track the connection between changes in visual acuity and spinal manipulative therapy (SMT).

- The authors noted that after SMT many patients stated that their vision has improved.

- In order to support this argument the authors decided to review all of the literature that tracks SMT with changes in oculomotor function, visual acuity, intraocular pressure and pupillary size.

- The complete literature available on spinal treatment and vision changed was searched, and it was discovered that from 1964 to 1992 there were 187 journal articles that described the experience of 187 patients who reported visual changes following cervical spin care.

- Gorman posits that improvements in eye conditions and vision are simply a side effect of the overall improved brain functioning caused by chiropractic adjustments.

## The prospective treatment of visual perception deficit by chiropractic spinal manipulation: a report on two juvenile patients

F. *The prospective treatment of visual perception deficit by chiropractic spinal manipulation: a report on two juvenile patients.* Stephens D., Gorman RF., Chiropractic Journal of Australia. 1996; 26:82-86.

- Case study of two pediatric patients: A 14-year old girl and an 8-year old girl who both suffered from tunnel vision (constricted visual fields). After seven visits (once a week) the 14 year old's visual acuity went from 20/50 in both eyes to 20/25 in both eyes. The 8-year old was 20/25 in both eyes before care and 20/25 right eye and 20/30 left eye after care.

**The step phenomenon in the glaucomatous recovery of vision with spinal manipulation: A report on two 13-year-olds treated together.**

G. *The step phenomenon in the glaucomatous recovery of vision with spinal manipulation: A report on two 13-year-olds treated together.* Stephens D, Gorman F, Bilton D. J Manip Physiol Ther 1997;20(9):628-633.

- Presents the theory of the "step phenomenon" which is the concept that gradual, step like improvements in visual function can occur after undergoing regular spinal adjustments.

- Study followed two 13-year-old cousins who suffered from diminished visual acuities and constricted visual fields.

**Bilateral simultaneous optic nerve dysfunction after pariorbital trauma: Recovery of vision in association with chiropractic spinal manipulation therapy.**

H. *Bilateral simultaneous optic nerve dysfunction after pariorbital trauma: Recovery of vision in association with chiropractic spinal manipulation therapy.* Stephens, D . Pollard, H., Bilton, D., Thomson, P., Gorman, RF. Journal of Manipulative & Physiological Therapeutics, Vol. 22, Issue 9, pp. 615–621 (1999).

- This is a study of 17 consecutive patients ranging in ages from 9-52 years of age, who all suffered from concentric narrowing of their visual fields. Typical symptoms included dizziness, blurred vision, fatigue, photophobia and headaches.

- 11 patients reported complete recovery of their visual fields and also the relief of their accompanying treatments.

- For example, one 21-year-old male patient had reported suffering from blurred vision, memory disturbance, postural hypertension and severe headaches for 7 months after suffering a head trauma.

- Following this trauma, a narrowing of that patient's visual fields were found and the patient received spinal care. After patient's first chiropractic treatment patient's headaches stopped, his dizziness decreased and memory improved. Following the second visit, patient's visual field returned to normal.

## Monocular scotoma and spinal manipulation: the step phenomenon.

1. *Monocular scotoma and spinal manipulation: the step phenomenon.* Gorman, RF Journal of Manipulative and Physiological Therapeutics 1996; 19:344-9.

- The objective of this study was to outline the case history of a 62-year-old male patient with scotoma vision of the right eye and a microvascular spasm of the optic nerve, who was treated with spinal manipulation.

- Patient received spinal manipulation treatment on an ongoing basis, which resolved the patient's scotoma. The rate of recovery of patient's scotoma was mapped via the use of a computerized static perimetry. The measurements from this mapping illustrated significant recovery occurring at each stage of the spinal manipulation treatment.

- The author posits that spinal manipulation affects the blood supply of the brain tissues localized areas, and a converse implication was presented that spinal derangement causes microvascular abnormalities.

- The author concluded that "Sspinal manipulation can affect the function of the optic nerve in some patients presumably by increasing vascular perfusion."

**Effects of a chiropractic adjustment on changes in pupillary diameter: a model for evaluating somatovisceral response.**

*J. Effects of a chiropractic adjustment on changes in pupillary diameter: a model for evaluating somatovisceral response.* Biggs L, Boone WR. Journal of Manipulative and Physiological Therapeutics, 1988; 11: 181-189.

- The relationship between a cervical chiropractic adjustment in subluxated vs. unsubluxated subjects, and autonomic response monitored as change in pupillary diameter was evaluated in 15 subjects.

- Pupillary diameter was shown to change significantly following manipulation in those shown to have a subluxation complex by a battery of chiropractic tests.

- Controls without subluxation were given a sham treatment (massage) to differentiate a placebo or nonspecific effect. They exhibited no pupillary change on follow-up.

## Study on cervical visual disturbance and its manipulative treatment.

K. *Study on cervical visual disturbance and its manipulative treatment.* Changjiand I, Yici W, Wenquin L et al. Journal of Traditional Chinese Medicine 1984 4:205.

- This is a report on 114 cases of patients with cervical spondylosis who reported associate visual disorders. Following manipulative treatment visual improvements were reported in 83% of these cases.

- Of the 54 cases followed up for a minimum of six months, 91% showed a stable therapeutic effect. Cases of blind eyes regaining vision were also included within the report.

## Monocular visual loss after closed head trauma: immediate resolution associated with spinal manipulation

L. *Monocular visual loss after closed head trauma: immediate resolution associated with spinal manipulation.* R. Frank Gorman. Journal of Manipulative and Physiological Therapeutics. Vol. 18, No.3, June 1995.

- Discusses the case history of a 9-year old patient who complained of blurred vision and headaches. Patient's visual fields were constricted and she also had a history of recurrent abdominal pain, headaches and "red eyes." The patient had two sessions with the author, who practiced spinal manipulation while the patient was under anesthesia.

- Author reported that "for a year after the spinal treatment, the patient had a much better demeanor and was generally free of troublesome headaches and ocular symptoms."

## Chiropractic adjustments and esophoria: a retrospective study and theoretical discussion.

M. *Chiropractic adjustments and esophoria: a retrospective study and theoretical discussion.* Schutte B, Teese H, Jamison J: J Aust Chiro Assoc Dec 1989 19(4): 126.

- Provides a retrospective review of 12 children with esophoria, which is a deviation of a visual axis towards that of the other eye when fusion is prevented.

- Author concluded that these patients may respond to cervical spine adjustments.

## The side effects of the chiropractic adjustment

N. *The side effects of the chiropractic adjustment.* Arno Burnier, D.C. Chiropractic Pediatrics Vol. 1 No. 4 May 1995.

- Provides the case history for a 17-year-old female who suffered from headaches and wore "coca cola" eyeglasses for nearsightedness.

- Patient presented the following vertebral subluxation: Axis posterior, D1/D2 PIR, D12/L1 Pl. The original adjustment is as follows: Meningeal contact on sacrum double notch, structural manual adjustment of D1/D2 in lateral flexion and extension, D12/L1 in extension and axis in extension supine with a spinous contact.

- Within three months of care, patient was symptom

free, no longer needing glasses. Results remained consistent for two years.

## The Treatment of Presumptive Optic-Nerve Ischemia by Spinal Manipulation.

O. *The Treatment of Presumptive Optic-Nerve Ischemia by Spinal Manipulation.* Gorman RF. J Manip Physiol Ther 1995;18(3):172-177. - A case report where a 62-year old male with a 1-week history of monocular visual defect experienced dramatic visual improvement after a week of spinal manipulation. - -- Author stated that "spinal manipulation can affect the function of the optic nerve in some patients presumably by increasing vascular perfusion."

## Monocular visual loss closed head trauma: immediate resolution associated with spinal manipulation.

P. *Monocular visual loss closed head trauma: immediate resolution associated with spinal manipulation.* R. Frank Gorman. Journal of Manipulative and Physiological Therapeutics. Vol. 18, No.3, June 1995.

-The author is a medical doctor investigating spinal care and it's relationship to vision, mental health, emotional wellness and overall health.

- Article focuses on the specific case of a 9-year old patient complaining of headaches and "red eyes".

- The author administered manipulation under anesthesia as part of the patient's treatment.

- Following two manipulations "For a year after the spinal treatment, the patient had a much better demeanor and was generally free of troublesome headaches and ocular symptoms.

- Hypotheses regarding the pathogenesis of this condition (visual problems and recovery after manipulation) is discussed.

## An observer's view of the treatment of visual perception by spinal manipulation. A survey of 16 patients

Q. *An observer's view of the treatment of visual perception by spinal manipulation. A survey of 16 patients.* Gorman RF. Sydney, Australia, 1991 (published privately).

- Four ophthalmologists examined 12 patients before and after spinal manipulation. In all cases the vision improved (either the visual field and /or visual acuity).

- Patient's following non-visual difficulties also improved: "spine hump straightening our, arm movement improved," "feels more positive and a lot happier. Does not wake up in the morning tired. More outgoing and talkative."

## Cortical blindness, cerebral palsy, epilepsy and recurring otitis media: A case study in chiropractic management.

R. *Cortical blindness, cerebral palsy, epilepsy and recurring otitis media: A case study in chiropractic management*. Amalu WC, Today's Chiropractic May/June 1998 pp.16-25.

- Case study about a 5-year-old boy with recurring middle-ear infections at one-month intervals who was diagnosed with cortical blindness (the eyes functioned properly but the vision center in the brain was damaged), cerebral palsy, epilepsy and severe brain damage, secondary to possible aborted crib death or viral encephalitis.

- His mother reported he had been a healthy child and "Two days following a well-child checkup with an inoculation," the child became "colicky" and developed a mild upper respiratory infection with fever and later became cyanotic, gasping for air and nonresponsive.

- A cranial CT scan showed cerebral edema, comparable with either an ischemic insult or sepsis. Child began to have seizures 24 hours later, diagnosed as severe hypoxemic encephalopathy, secondary to possible SIDS or vital encephalitis.

- Patient's health issues may have been vaccine related injury, especially since cerebral edema is a sign of vaccine damage. Also encephalopathy has been noticed in the medical literature as a possible reaction to the DTP inoculation. Upon discussion with the author of this paper it was learned that the medical personnel refused to acknowledge or even consider possible vaccine injury.

- At the time of patient's first chiropractic visit he was having 30 grand mal and complex seizures a day and otitis media once per month. Patient was unable to walk, communicate and was non-responsive. He made a constant loud vocal drone and almost constant writhing torsocephalic motions.

- Patient underwent chiropractic management that consisted of correction (adjustment) of C1 vertebrae.

- Patient's mother noted that he had his first good-night sleep in weeks.

- After the 2nd adjustment, patient's seizures reduced to 10/day, vocal drone became a quiet intermittent moan and he began to clap his hands.

- During the next week patient had became more alert, sitting up and looking around, and responded to sounds. Seizures decreased to 5/day. Pupillary reflexes returned to normal, almost all writhing motions had ceased, ears were clear of effusion. By the 3rd week grand mal seizures had stopped and he was sleeping through the night.

- By end of the fifth week of chiropractic treatment an ophthalmologist noted a drastic improvement in central field vision. Seizures reduced to three per day, saying more words and improved fine motor coordination.

- Over the next 10 months improvement continued. All epileptic symptoms disappeared and the neurologist declared him non-epileptic. Patient's vision improved to the point where he was prescribed glasses, and he remained free from ear infections.

## Case report: spinal strain and visual perception deficit

S. *Case report: spinal strain and visual perception deficit.* Gorman RF, Anderson RL, Hilton D, Favoloro RJ, Pittorino AJ. Chiropractic J. of Australia 1994: 24: 131-134

- Following a motor vehicle accident, a 33-year-old male experienced an overall "burning" feeling, difficulty in breathing, vertigo on standing, fatigue, irritability, pain in the right wrist, sore eyes, and blurred vision. X-rays and EKG were normal. Patient also had tunnel vision.

- Following spinal care patient's symptoms completely disappeared.

# Conclusion

Popular media likes to scare viewers into thinking chiropractic care is dangerous and can cause strokes or break your neck. Chiropractic adjustments, if done correctly, have an amazing effect on the body as has been shown in the above studies.

I hope you have enjoyed this fact-filled book. If you haven't read the previous two books in the series, you can get them at relaxtoclarity.com or on amazon.com.

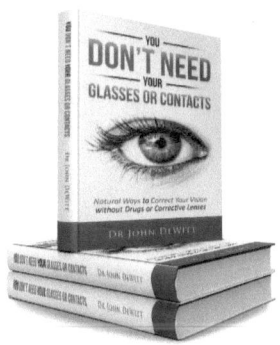
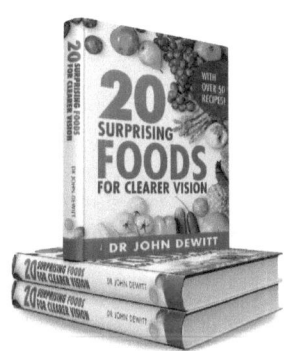

*Dr John DeWitt*

# CHIROPRACTIC CARE FOR CLEARER VISION 127

RelaxToClarity.com

Made in United States
Troutdale, OR
06/05/2024

20343080R00076